Sleep Apnea
Symptoms, diagnosis and treatment

Garth Howell

CONTENTS

1   What is Sleep Apnea   Pg 1

2   Sleep Apnea Categories   Pg 3

3   Definitions   Pg 5

4   Symptoms and Signs   Pg 6

5   Diagnosis   Pg 9

6   Treatment   Pg 15

7   Problems   Pg 25

8   Provent Technology   Pg 29

9   Conclusion   Pg 30

10 References   Pg 32

Garth Howell

What is Sleep Apnea

Sleep Apnea is a medical condition of which there are a great number of sufferers, but unfortunately many cases go undiagnosed, and this in turn creates associated problems for the sufferer such as irritability, weight gain, diabetes heart problems. It is a serious condition that can and does cause serious illness, loss of quality of life and in some cases fatality.

Sleep is an important part of our lives and is driven by natural brain activity. Unless you have adequate deep sleep each night your mind and body will never feel refreshed. Most people need about 8 hours of sleep per night of which about 15%-25% should be of the deepest sleep known, as slow wave sleep, in order to be fully rested and refreshed.

Put simply, sleep apnea is a condition where the sufferer temporarily stops breathing whilst asleep. or in some cases the breathing is very shallow. The interruptions to the breathing can be a few times every hour or can be many, and the shallow breathing can sometimes go on for several minutes. I have come across sufferers who stop breathing in excess of 80 times per hour. After the event the sufferer usually will let out a loud snort as if they are choking and they return to normal breathing until the next episode.

Understandably, this constant disturbance prevents a good nights sleep being experienced by the sufferer and they tend to wake up feeling tired and sometimes with a headache. This interruption also means that the sufferer due to lack of sleep will feel tired all day.

Diagnosis is not that easy, as it is unlikely to be discovered during a routine medical examination. The sufferer may be aware of having a disturbed nights sleep, but would not necessarily put that down to anything abnormal. A partner may know you are a loud snorer but wouldn't think anything about it other than being disturbed too. Most peple would not usually consult their doctor about their disturbed sleep.

There are many millions of people suffering from sleep apnea throughout the world but as yet it is undiagnosed. Some say it could be over 1 in 5. It does tend to affect you more if you are overweight, and it is a condition that more men suffer from than women. It is also more likely to affect you if the airways in your throat are narrow for some reason, and it is likely to affect you more as you get older. Sleep apnea can affect children, particularly children with enlarged tonsils.

If you are a smoker you have a greater risk off developing sleep apnea and also if you have high blood pressure.

Sleep Apnea Categories

There are several types of sleep apnea, the most common type and the type we will be concentrating on in this book is known as Obstructive Sleep Apnea. In effect what happens with Obstructive Sleep Apnea (OSA) is that whilst you are sleeping you are relaxed and your throat muscles collapse cuasing an interruption in breathing.

Another type of sleep apnea is known as Central Sleep Apnea (CSA) and this condition is different from OSA as the muscles controlling breathing receive incorrect signals from the brain and the third, a combination of both the other conditions.

Obstructive Sleep Apnea

With OSA whilst you are asleep several things happen:-

1. The throat muscles collapse inwards

2. You try to breathe but due to the airway being blocked you are unsuccessful

3. As a consequence of above the level of oxygen in the blood drops.

4. The brain then signals to the body to take a breath to re-oxygenate the blood and as a consequence you gasp for air.

5. You will not necessarily wake up during these episodes even though you will probably make a snorting sound as you struggle to get air.

The diagnosis of OSA is normally made when you have 5 or more episodes as described above happening per hour.

Central Sleep apnea

Central Sleep Apnea is a rarer condition than OSA and accounts for fewer than 5% of sleep apnea cases. It occurs when the brain does not send correct signals to the airway muscles to allow you to breathe normally. As oxygen levels decrease you may well wake up. Central sleep apnea may occur as the result of a heart attack or stroke or some other medical conditions and sleeping at high altitudes may also create an occurrence.

Mixed Sleep Apnea

This is a combination of the above types inasmuch that sufferers show signs of OSA but when a persistent positive air pressure is applied they then demonstrate signs of Central Sleep Apnea. It is recognised as a distinct type of sleep apnea and has individual recognised characteristics. This publication does not seek to deal with this condition in detail.

Definitions

There are couple of terms used regularly in conjunction with sleep apnea and it is important that they are understood.

Apnea

An apnea is where the throat muscles and surrounding tissue relaxes sufficuently to cause a total blockage of the airway for a period of 10 seconds or more.

Hypopnea

A hypopnea occurs when there is a partial blockage of the airway for 10 seconds or morem causing a 50% or more reduction in airflow.

Symptoms and Signs of Sleep Apnea

We have touched on the main symptom and indicator which is the gasping for air and snoring but there are others. The snoring is normally helped by sleeping on your side and when sleeping on your back the snoring can get much worse. It may not occur every night but over time it is likely to become more frequent and the snoring may be louder.

As your sleep has been disturbed it is likely that you will end up being tired throughout the day, in fact you may never feel as if you have enjoyed a really good nights settled sleep. The result is that you may need to sleep during the day, particularly if you are not involved in any activity. The result of this can be dangerous as it is possible that you could end up having an accident, not good, particularly if you are driving.

There other signs that you may be experiencing the symptoms of sleep apnea:-

1. Waking up with a dry throat

2. Having a headache first thing in the morning on a regular basis.

3. Difficulty with concentrating on tasks.

4. Memory loss.

5. Being irritable, short tempered, moody and experiencing a change in your temperament.

6. You may find that you have to urinate more frequently, particularly during the evening and night.

One of the functions of the muscles in the throat is to ensure that the airways are kept open to enable you to breathe. If these muscles relax however the airway becomes blocked, and makes breathing difficult, or causes it to cease due to air being unable to pass into your lungs.

The sleep apnea suffer may have a smaller than normal airway in the mouth and throat.

The tongue and throat muscles are more relaxed than they should be.

If you are overweight then there will be more fatty tissue in the throat and neck area than normal. This can thicken in the windpipe wall and cause the windpipe to narrow making it difficult for air to pass.

A combination of relaxed muscles and fatty tissue in the neck complicates the situation further and can really make breathing difficult.

As people get older the signals from the brain may not function in as well as they did and the throat muscles are not kept as stiff.

If your airways are blocked or constricted then you are very likely to snore loudly as you sleep and you will not be aware of it taking place due to the fact that you are sleeping.

As you are not breathing properly there will be low oxygen levels in the blood, which in turn will disturb your sleep further. The muscles in your windpipe will tighten up and so cause the airway to open again, and you will breath normally. The muscles will then relax and you start snoring and snorting once again. It's a vicious cycle.

Stress hormones will be released as the body is not in harmony with itself, and these can cause you to have elevated blood pressure which increases the chance of a heart attack, stroke, irregular heartbeat or even heart failure.

If the condition is not treated it is very likely to lead to the sufferer gaining weight and as a consequence developing diabetes.

The Diagnosis of Sleep Apnea

If you are suffering from any of the signs that are associated with sleep apnea sufferers then you should speak to your Doctor about it. Tiredness can be caused by a number of reasons, one of them being an under active thyroid. If you snore and sleep with a partner I am sure you will have been informed about it. Tell your Doctor who, if they suspect that you could be a sleep apnea sufferer or just want to rule sleep apnea out of the equation, will refer you to have a sleep study done, probably at a specialist sleep clinic. The sleep clinic should be able to confirm a diagnosis.

If you are referred, I urge you to ensure that you take it as the risks associated with the condition are great, and should not be ignored.

When you visit the sleep clinic you will be asked a number of questions which will form the prelude to the sleep study proper. Some typical questions are:-

The time you went to bed the previous night?

The time you woke up in the morning?

How long you slept for the previous night?

How many times did you wake up?

How long did it take you to fall asleep?

What medications you took before going to bed?

Did you feel refreshed when you woke up or still sleepy?

How many caffeine drinks do you consume over the course of a day?

The number of alcoholic drinks you consume in the course of a day?

Did you have any day time naps?

If yes, how many and for how long?

Were you awake or feeling sleepy through the day?

Did you suffer from any morning headaches?

The practitioner carrying out the tests will also check your blood pressure, weigh you and will most likely check collar size.

The Epworth Sleepiness Test

The practitioner will also carry out the Epworth test which is a test to determine your daytime sleepiness. The test is so named as it was developed by Dr. Murray Johns at the Epworth Hospital in Melbourne Australia. It is quite simple to carry out and asks you what appear on the surface to be some rather odd questions. You requested to work out how the questions would have affected you on the scale as follows:-

0 = no chance of dozing

1 = small chance of dozing

2 = moderate chance of dozing

3 = high chance of dozing

The questions are regarding the following situations:-

Sitting and reading

Watching TV

Sitting inactive in a public place e.g. theatre or a meeting

As a passenger in a car for an hour without a break

Lying down to rest in the afternoon (when circumstances permit)

Sitting and talking to someone

Sitting quietly for a lunch without alcohol

In a car while stopped for a few minutes in traffic.

After answering the questions using the scoring as outlined above the scores are added up.

If the score is high then it advisable not to drive or use dangerous machinery until the cause has been established.

The score doesn't demonstrate the presence of sleep apnea or any other sleep related problems as there are several issues that could cause daytime sleepiness. It does however show that further investigation is required to find out the cause of the problem.

The Sleep Study

The sleep study is carried out in a sleep centre clinic and the main investigation is known as a Polysomnography and you will need to stay in overnight for this test. Normally you turn up early evening with an overnight bag. You then have various electrodes connected to the face scalp and just above your lip. Bands will go round your abdomen and chest. You will also have sensors placed on your legs and there will also be a finger sensor attached. A microphone will also be attached.

The following tests are then carried out.

An electro-encephalography (EEG) which monitors your brain waves.

An electromyography to monitor muscle tone.

The movements of your chest and abdomen (thoracoabdominal).

Your oronasal airflow will be measured i.e. airflow in the mouth and the nose.

Heart rate and blood oxygen levels (pulse oximetry).

Electrocardiogram (ECG) to measure your heart.

Sound and video recording will also be carried out to check how loudly you snore and how much you move.

The signals from the test will be monitored by specialist sleep nurses during the early part of the night. If Obstructive Sleep Apnea symptoms are noticed then you will be given some CPAP (continuous positive airway pressure) treatment where you will be fitted with a mask covering both the nose and mouth where a constant pressure of air is applied to keep the airways open.

Once this test has been carried out the clinic will have a good idea as to whether you are suffering from OSA, the severity and how they should be treating it.

Home Study

You may be offered a home study as an alternative to an overnight stay at a clinic. This can be more convenient but it will involve you visiting the sleep clinic to have instruction on how to use the equipment which you will then take home. The equipment will also need to be returned the following day and the results downloaded and analysed.

The portable equipment to carry out the test includes:-

A breathing sensor.

Sensors to monitor your heart rate.

Oxygen sensors which are attached to a finger and a band around the chest.

This does not supply as much information as the Polysomnography but in many cases is enough to enable the correct diagnosis of OSA to be made.

The severity of OSA is measured by the number apnea and hypopnea episodes occur per hour and are measured using the AHI (Apnea Hypopnea Index)

A score of 5-14 episodes per hour is rated as mild

15-30 episodes per hour are rated as moderate

Over 30 is rated as severe.

If the AHI is below 10 then you would not normally be considered as having a disorder.

A sleep study appears to be quite a scary and stressful activity but in reality there is nothing to worry about and it most certainly is not a painful experience.

Treatment for Sleep Apnea

There are several ways of approaching the treatment of sleep apnea. Lifestyle adjustments can be made which can help alleviate the symptoms, and reduce the number of hypopnea's or apnea's occurring whilst you are sleeping.

If you are overweight then losing some pounds should help considerably.

If you are a smoker it is advisable to stop as smoking does not help the condition.

Drink alcohol within the recommended guidelines.

It may also help to sleep on your side rather than your back. This may reduce the symptoms although it will not eliminate them or prevent the condition.

For mild cases it may be enough to make simple lifestyle changes but if the condition is severe then you will probably be treated with a continuous positive airway pressure (CPAP). With this treatment you use a mask which covers both the mouth and the nose attached to a machine which supplies a constant pressure of air to help with your breathing by ensuring that the airways are kept open. You use this at night whilst you sleep.

The early versions of the CPAP machine were known to have some side effects such as a dry or sore throat, dry nasal passages and, in some cases, nose bleeds. These symptoms have been reduced somewhat by fitting the machine with a humidifier which adds some moisture to the air. This certainly does help relieve that problem.

Some CPAP machines also start working at a low pressure which gradually builds over 20 minutes before reaching the optimum pressure set for you by your sleep clinic. This is to allow you to drift off to sleep more easily. Some even have a small heater which ensures that warm air is supplied. This can be very useful in cold atmospheres.

There are some other possible side effects of using a CPAP machine which may be experienced by the user.

The mask can be uncomfortable or can slip

This is quite common and during the early days of using a CPAP machine I am sure that most people find the mask, attached to a machine via a long pipe quite intrusive. Once however you have managed to get some good nights sleep you will find that you feel better and you will get used to the mask. You will also tend to move around less while sleeping. If the mask moves out of position it can help to just reset the machine to start up and let the pressure build again.

The masks are extremely well designed and this helps it to reseal.

Nasal congestion

This too is a common side effect which is helped by having a CPAP with a humidifier but if it continues you may need to seek help to alleviate the congestion and the same goes for any difficulty breathing through the nose.

Headaches and possible ear pain

These too are a possible side effect to watch out for if using a CPAP machine

Stomach pain and flatulence

These too can be experienced due to air getting into the stomach.

If you experience any of the above or are concerned then either speak to your sleep clinic or your Doctor who should be able to help and advise.

Oral Appliances

Oral appliances known as Mandibular Responding Splints (MRS) have a use in treating sleep apnea. It is a dental appliance similar to a gum shield which is worn in the mouth whilst you sleeping. It is designed to push the jaw and tongue slightly forward which increases the space at the back of the throat enough to maintain a clear and open airway through which you can breathe.

The MRS needs to made for you by an orthodontist who will take impressions of your teeth and jaw. The MRS once in use should last about 18 months before it needs replacing. If you have crowns, caps or bridges in your moth your dentist should be able to advise as you do want them to be put under undue stress.

Surgery

There are surgical procedures that can be carried out to alleviate OSA, however they are usually used as a last resort as they are not as effective as the CPAP which is generally regarded as the gold standard treatment.

Various surgical options may be considered as if you have a deviated nasal septum, tonsils which are enlarged or a small lower jaw.

Other surgical treatments can involve the removal of tonsils and adenoids, the removal of excess tissue in the throat to widen the airway (uvupalatopharyngoplasty) and even a trachostomy where a tube is inserted into the neck to allow you to breathe.

This section is just to make the reader aware that there are medical procedures available for some cases. This publication will not go into any more detail regarding surgery as it is beyond the remit of the author, who believes that advice from qualified medical practitioners who have the required level of expertise should be sought.

CPAP Equipment

The CPAP machine cones in various types but they are designed to supply air at a pressure sufficient to maintain an open airway to enable you to breathe whilst sleeping.

The Various types may be categorised as follows:-

CPAP (continuous positive air pressure) machine which supplies air at a constant pressure which is put in place when the machine is set up. The higher the AHI then the greater the pressure will be required to keep the airway open. Some machines are fitted with a ramp facility where the pressure gradually increases over the first 20 minutes or so to allow you to sleep before it is blowing at full pressure.

APAP (Automatic positive air pressure)

This is similar to the CPAP but supplies enough air to keep the airway open on a breath by breath basis. This ensures that you always have the ideal pressure for you.

OSA sufferers often prefer to us an APAP machine, finding it more comfortable.. APAP machines can operate like a CPAP blowing at a constant pressure but a CPA cannot be made to operate like an APAP.

With an APAP the machine is set to blow at the highest pressure to maintain a free airway.

BIPAP Machine

The BIPAP machine is also sometimes referred to as a bi level machine or VPAP is a variation on the CPAP but it supplies to pressures of air, one when the user inhales and a different pressure on exhalation. The pressures are set by the medical practitioner when the machine is personalised for the user.

The Bipap machine is useful in treating sleep apnea in people who may also have other conditions such a congestive heart failure and certain lung disorders. Certain tests are usually carried out to assess for suitability to using a Bipap. A respiratory test is likely to be carried out to measure lung capacity. A forced vital capacity test may also be carried out which will measure the depth of breath that a person is able to take.

This area requires qualified medical examination and testing and only a medical practitioner can advise on the individuals suitability or not for using a Bipap machine.

The Bipap can also be obtained in an auto version which responds to each individual inhalation and exhalation.

Masks

The face mask is an extremely important part of the equipment. Once the diagnosis has been made and the required pressure established to maintain an open airway it will be necessary to turn your attention as to how you will be connected to the PAP machine. You will be fitted with a mask which will be connected to the PAP machine by a length of flexible tubing. The most important factors surrounding the mask are that it is not too intrusive and is comfortable and you have minimal air leakage from around the seals whilst in use. Any leakage will quite naturally affect the pressure of air being supplied and can render the PAP less effective.

The straps holding the mask to your face do not have to be too tight as if they are the mask will be uncomfortable and you will be more likely to get air leaking from the seals. The headgear must neither be too tight or loose but must feel snug. The straps holding the mask have adjusters which once set stay put so you do not have to adjust the straps each time you put on the mask. Quick release clips are also provided to enable the user to remove or put on the mask with a minimum of difficulty.

Masks come in different sizes to suit all faces. If the mask is too large it will be more likely to leak air so select a mask which is a snug fit.

Various types of masks are available to suit all users:-

Full Face Masks

Full face masks cover quite a large area of your face from the bridge of your nose to your chin or just above it. These allow the user to breathe through the nose and mouth and are useful for people who tend to breathe through the mouth.

Nasal Cushion Masks

Nasal cushion masks are triangular in shape and go from the bridge of the nose to just above your upper lip. A chinstrap can be provided to stop your mouth from dropping open whist sleeping. They do not work well with people who have a deviated septum or for those who have sinus problems. A chinstrap can be provided to stop your mouth from dropping open whist sleeping.

Nasal Pillow Masks

The nasal pillow mask feeds the air directly through your nasal passages. They are good for people who would feel claustrophobic if using a full face mask. They can work well if you like to read with your mask on as they permit you to wear glasses but not so good if you move around a lot or prefer sleeping on your side.

They do not have any contact with your face but using small silicone nipples rest on the perimeter of your nostrils. They too do not work well with people who have a deviated septum or for those who have sinus problems.

Hybrid Mask

This type of mask combines an oral mask and a nasal pillow mask and covers the nostrils down to below the bottom lip and just above the chin. They work well for those people who really need a face mask but find it claustrophobic.

Oral Mask

The oral mask is really only for consideration if all other mask types have been found to be unsuitable. They rest between the gums and the lips and you breathe through your mouth.

We are designed to breathe through our noses and as such are equipped to filter bacteria and breathing through the mouth means that these systems are bypassed. This therefore leaves the wearer of this type of mask prone to picking up infection.

Problems Incurred by PAP Users

It is quite normal to experience some problems when you first start using a PAP machine and wearing a mask.

Claustrophobia

It may help if you feel claustrophobic with a mask to do some practice before you use it. Try the mask during the day, firstly by just holding it to your face without straps just to get used to the feel of it. Then attach the straps and try it and finally switch the machine on.

If you are still having problems then try relaxation exercises. If you can learn to relax you may well find it easier. It is understandable that initially you may feel embarrassed about wearing a mask but over time that should pass.

It could also be that the mask is the wrong size or just badly set up. In any event talk to your medical professional who should be able to offer assistance.

Difficulty with tolerating air being blown.

This is a very common problem and getting used to the air being blown takes some doing as it is unnatural. Using the ramp feature should help you get to sleep as the air blown is very gently initially and gradually builds up. By the time it is at the maximum pressure you should be asleep.

If you are still having problems then talk to your medical professional about the possibility of using a APAP machine which just responds when needed or even perhaps a Bipap machine.

Stuffy, dry nose or nosebleeds

This is another common problem which may be help by using a humidifier. Also using saline nasal sprays can be effective in keeping the nasal passages moist and avoiding infection.

Another option which can help is to have a humidifier attached to the machine to maintain a supply of moist air as you sleep.

If your mask is leaking this too can dry out your nose.

Leaky mask or pressure sores

It is important that the mask seals properly otherwise you will not be receiving air at the correct pressure. Air may too get into your eyes causing them to be dry or runny.

It is important that the straps are properly tensioned and the pads are in the correct position and are in good condition.

It may also be worth checking with your healthcare professional that the mask is the correct size or perhaps another type could be more suitable for you.

The noise

Modern machines are usually very quiet and emit little, if any sound. If there is noise then check the filters and tubes for obstruction. You will also find there is obtrusive noise if there are any leaks of air around the mask so ensure that the mask seals correctly.

If you are still unsettled by the sound then you may like to see if earplugs help but this should not be necessary.

Dry mouth

This may be caused by you breathing through your mouth or sleeping with your mouth open. If this is the case then a chinstrap may help to keep your mouth shut whilst you sleep. As with problems associated with a dry nose you may find that a humidifier will help.

Summary

You will find that over time the using of a PAP machine will get easier and you will be more comfortable about using it. You should gradually start to feel much better as hopefully you are getting a good nights sleep. This should have a positive effect on your life and for those around you. If you are not feeling tired all the time it is likely that you will be happier in yourself, have more energy and be less irritable. When you are used to using a PAP machine you will find that the sensation of slow, regular breathing that you will experience to be well worth the effort of familiarising yourself with using it. It is easy to say but just try to be relaxed about it.

If you maintain the equipment correctly and have reviews with your healthcare professional you will hopefully discover that having had the diagnosis of sleep apnea made has a positive effect on your life.

Provent Technology

There is a fairly new treatment for sleep apnea known as Provent Therapy which is claimed to be an alternative treatment for sleep apnea. It is also claimed that studies have been made which demonstrate significant improvement in the symptoms of OSA, reduction in snoring and also a reduction in daytime sleepiness.

The device is placed just inside the nostrils and held in place by a light hypoallergenic adhesive. It works by allowing you to inhale normally, but there is a one way valve in the device which on exhalation creates an expiaratory positive airway pressure which keeps the airway open. The device is small and is disposable which makes it very convenient, particularly if you are travelling as it avoids having to carry a bulky CPAP.

I understand the device is FDA approved and clinically proven although the writer has no personal experience of the device.

Provent technology is currently available in the United States, Australia, Hong Kong, Malaysia and New Zealand and I would imagine that it will, over time be available in other countries.

I understand that where it is available it is well tolerated by users and has a high degree of acceptance.

Conclusion

Sleep apnea is a dangerous condition and the writer is a sufferer. I use CPAP and whilst I found it difficult to begin with, have learnt to live with it and have adjusted my lifestyle accordingly. I now find that the sleep that I get to be excellent and there are times when my breathing becomes very slow and deep and most refreshing.

I use a full face mask and have found that it is essential to have it fully sealed on the face. If it is not then air will leak and you end up with a blast of air onto your face and the airflow does not settle to a slow balanced shhhh, just sufficient just to keep the airway open. The straps holding the mask in place do not have to be tight, in fact having it too tight can affect the seal. If correctly tensioned and positioned the mask can be quite comfortable.

To avoid nasal congestion I sometimes put a few drops of Olbas Oil which is an oil composed of scents such as menthol and I find the air coming in is then very fragrant.

The CPAP is currently regarded as the gold standard treatment with an almost 100% of success rate of respite from those who use it. I would urge any OSA sufferers who read this book to keep going with the

CPAP although it may be difficult to begin with. Once you have conquered it you will feel so much better. I was diagnosed with OSA by an anaesthetist who was interviewing me before some surgery. His words were "get tested and if you have OSA get treated. It will change your life"

I got treated and he was correct, so don't be afraid, just keep going.

I wish you the very best of luck. I do hope that you manage to get your OSA under control, whatever method you use.

References

References for provent

1. Berry RB, Kryger MH, Massie CA. A novel nasal expiratory positive airway pressure (EPAP) device for the treatment of obstructive sleep apnea:
a randomized controlled trial. Sleep. 2011;34:479-485.

2. Walsh JK, Griffin KS, Forst EH, et al. A convenient expiratory positive airway pressure nasal device for the treatment of sleep apnea in patients
non-adherent with continuous positive airway pressure. Sleep Med. 2011;12:147-152.

3. Rosenthal L, Massie CA, Dolan DC, Loomas B, Kram J, Hart RW. A multicenter, prospective study of a novel nasal EPAP device in the treatment
of obstructive sleep apnea: efficacy and 30-day adherence. J Clin Sleep Med. 2009;5:532-537.

4. Kryger MH, Berry RB, Massie CA. Long-term use of a nasal expiratory positive airway pressure (EPAP) device as a treatment for obstructive
sleep apnea (OSA). J Clin Sleep Med. 2011;7:449-453.

www.ingramcontent.com/pod-product-compliance
Lightning Source LLC
Chambersburg PA
CBHW050353290526
45785CB00006B/2753